Gone In *60* Minutes

LISA GAWTHORNE

**Grosvenor House
Publishing Limited**

Lisa Gawthorne is hereby identified as author of this
work in accordance with Section 77 of the Copyright, Designs
and Patents Act 1988

The book cover picture is copyright to Lisa Gawthorne

This book is published by
Grosvenor House Publishing Ltd
28-30 High Street, Guildford, Surrey, GU1 3EL.
www.grosvenorhousepublishing.co.uk

A CIP record for this book
is available from the British Library

ISBN 978-1-78148-770-9

Authors Disclaimer

This book is intended as a reference volume only, not as a medical manual. The information given here is designed to help you make informed decisions about your health. It is not intended as a substitute for any treatment that may have been prescribed by your doctor. Results will vary depending on the individual and it is always recommended to consult your doctor before starting any dietary, fitness or supplement plan. If you suspect you have a medical problem, it is recommended that you seek competent medical help. It is advised that the readers take full responsibility for their safety and know their limits. Before practising any exercises in this book, be sure that your equipment is well-maintained and do not take risks beyond your level of experience, aptitude, training and fitness. In summary – know your limits and don't be silly!

Poliquin Performance Centre Disclaimer

The foregoing book contains only the opinions and beliefs of the author which are not necessarily the opinions or beliefs of Poliquin Performance Center 2, LLC. The information contained in this book is based on the author's unique body analysis and experiences, and individual results are likely to vary. Because the Poliquin system is customized to each particular person's unique body analysis, the foregoing should not in any way be used as a substitute for the advice of or a relationship with a certified Poliquin trainer. Poliquin has not compensated the author in any way for the foregoing book. The book is not intended and should not be construed to claim that any Poliquin product can be used to diagnose, treat, cure, mitigate or prevent any disease; these statements have not been evaluated by the Food and Drug Administration.

"The fight is won or lost far away from witnesses – behind the lines, in the gym, and out there on the road, long before I dance under those lights."

Muhammad Ali

To all the Earth's Athletes.
New, old and yet to be.

Contents

Acknowledgements

The people who helped make this undertaking possible know who they are but I would like to take this opportunity to thank a few key individuals for their continued guidance and support. In particular:

James Slomka at Primal Health - for putting me through the gruelling weekly fitness sessions and recognising my constant hunger for rapid results.

My family – for putting up with my antisocial behaviour and my "Bob Cratchit" ways.

Karl Morris - for letting the world see his "before" photos online at www.gonein60minutes.co.uk.

Grosvenor Publishing - for their constant advice and help.

Michael Palmer Fitness Photography – for his uniquely creative vision.

Sweaty Betty clothing - for providing me with cutting edge fitness attire.

Formby Hall Golf Resort & Spa - for providing the studio as the backdrop for the web site exercises.

Heather Pearson at 1body4life - for healing my tendonitis with the magical ART®

Adam Slater at I-Design - for bringing my ideas to life.

Finally thanks to all my friends who gave feedback on the progress of the book and web site.

1

Gym Jargon Made Easy

ART – Active Release Techniques - a patented, state of the art soft tissue system/movement based massage technique that treats problems with muscles, tendons, ligaments, fascia and nerves.

Barbell = Long slim bar that is used to slide weighted discs on to for weighted movements.

BCAA = Branched Chain Amino Acids – The essential amino acids shown to improve performance, protect against muscle loss, decrease post workout soreness and stimulate protein synthesis.

Compound Exercises = A type of exercise that works a group of muscles in the body e.g. Chest press which works most of the upper body muscles.

DIM = Diindolylmethane – a natural supplement that has been shown to help balance oestrogen.

Dumbbell = Individual weight.

EFA's = Essential Fatty Acids.

HIIT = High intensity interval training.

Isometric Moves = A movement where muscles are tensed in one position without moving e.g. The Plank.

Isolation Exercises = An exercise that works a particular muscle group e.g. Bicep Curl which focuses on the parts of the bicep muscle.

LPS = Liverpool Pembroke Sefton.

Rep = The number of actual times you perform a single exercise.

Set = The number of times you repeat your reps.

SVT = Supraventricular Tachycardia – A disturbance of heart rhythm caused by rapid electrical activity in the upper part of the heart.

PT = Personal Trainer.

Tabata = High exercise intensity based on 20 seconds of effort (repetitions) followed by 10 seconds rest and this is repeated for 8 cycles.

Preface

It's October 2007 and I am lying on a bed in the cardiothoracic theatre at Broad Green Hospital. Morphine has been administered and it's time to have a radio frequency heart ablation. Before you check the front cover to make sure you're reading the right book let me share some more information with you. During 2007 I suffered two SVT attacks both of which sent my heart racing above 200 beats per minute and before you ask, I hadn't drank a few too many Red Bulls, this was a genetic health problem I had inherited from my poor mother who had spent many years being fanned down with a tea towel by my father and who after numerous years of being on medication and even a trip to the Intensive care unit at Ormskirk Hospital also had the same operation as myself. Watching your own heart on a plasma screen as a medical team lace wires from the top of your leg to your chest is up there as one of life's most surreal moments.

I had always been active and always been a member of a gym since early college days so it came as a bit of a shock to learn that my heart had an "extra piece" that was simply not needed and this extra piece was causing a "short circuit" of electricity. Learning that was daunting enough but then finding out that that extra piece was going to be "burnt off" was even harder to take. A few hours after the successful operation, I presented the doctors with an unusual question (so they told me), of how long it would be before I could start training again. Most people are thinking at this stage about recuperation and relaxation but I had a training plan to follow and races to enter! Although I would not recommend this, two days later I was slowly lifting weights whilst carefully monitoring my heart with a chest strap and wrist monitor. A week later I started running despite the slight pain at the top of my leg from the surgery which only served to make me strangely more determined to get better! Six weeks later I ran in the National Cross Country Championships with the biggest smile on my face, won a sponsor and made the front page of the local papers, ahead of the local football star Mr Steven Gerrard!

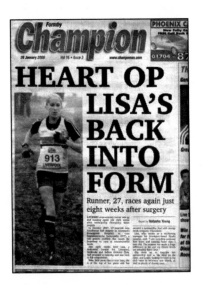

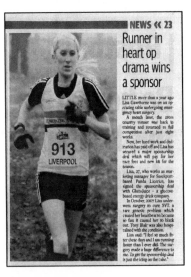

I had suffered, I had conquered and all that mattered to me now was my recovery plan. The reason I mention this whole experience is that I hope having gone through this trauma and sharing those moments with you, it will allow you to see that I came out the other end stronger and that any doubts you may have about what you can and can't do in your potential world of fitness may start to evaporate. You can get over almost anything if you are focused and determined enough. Physical exercise was the greatest sanctum to escape any worry and relax the mind back then and it's still the case today – it's my tonic, it runs through my veins, I can't imagine life without it and I enjoy it almost as much as baked beans!

After a few years of competitive running and gym going, I was doing ok – but *just ok* wasn't good enough and I wanted to make improvements in strength, speed, body tone and definition. After vetting the lists of local PTs I found one who was perfect in terms of his regime, his way of teaching and his educational background and knowledge on Charles Poliquin supplementation. James Slomka, a certified personal trainer has a BSC in Sports Science and Football and has completed the Poliquin™ BioSignature Modulation course. We have been working together for well over a year now and the results have been phenomenal. Like many people who work out in gyms or who run a lot, I was overdoing the cardio and this caused a plateau in fitness levels as well as muscle wastage. It was a hard lesson to learn and one of the most difficult things I have done but cutting down the cardio and picking up the weights has been the foundation to my most successful race season in my running history as well as adding tone and definition to all major muscle groups for achieving that classic athletic look I had always wanted but never managed to achieve. I have learned that I couldn't have done this on my own as I was getting nowhere fast. I now train each week with James at Primal Health to maintain all the hard work. It's the hardest hour of the week but I wouldn't have it any other way having seen the improvements in strength, stamina and body tone and the ever decreasing body fat.

Eating the right foods, taking the right supplements and being in the right state of mind have all had a big part to play in it and whilst each dimension along with the fitness aspect can be a minefield of information, this book will take each part and cover it in an easy to understand format so that you don't have to read the piles of books and magazines on fitness that I did.

I have drawn upon my knowledge of working in the health food industry, operating in the world of competitive athletics, being a lifelong gym member with access to a Poliquin Certified

Personal Trainer – bringing it altogether with learning's from multiple fitness and nutrition books and magazines to make this book happen.

So what are you waiting for, turn the page and in 60 minutes you will have all the answers you need to achieve that dream body.

Happy Days.

Lisa

CHAPTER 1 – WORKING OUT

Cardio makes you fat?!

If I was to tell you that your tiring long hour of cardio in your gym was making you fat, you would probably think I had lost leave of my senses because you're thinking if you come off a machine feeling exhausted or sweating, it can't be making you fat right? Well just before you settle for my word on it, why don't you type into google "cardio makes you fat" and see what is being said on the topic because although controversial and probably not what you want to hear if that's the way you have been working out, there is an increasing amount of evidence that says it could be the case.

One of the most famous and well documented speakers on this topic is Charles Poliquin – the world's greatest strength trainer and he has a whole army of Poliquin instructors who believe and teach the same premise in gyms around the globe. Keith Alpert his fitness colleague also teaches the same premise[1]. This is based on the formula that weight sessions are the key to sculpting the body, increasing the metabolism and reducing body fat whilst long sessions of flat cardio reduce muscle tone and stress the body in a way that increases cortisol levels which can make you fat! Not only that but Poliquin states that long sessions of cardio stress the body in a way that increases inflammation and can lower insulin sensitivity due to exposure to "dirty electricity" on machines and advises that strength training is incorporated into fitness routines to combat the negative effects of aerobic exercise[2].

9

What is Cortisol?

Cortisol is a stress hormone that has been linked to increases in weight gain and it eats away at muscle tissue – we have all heard at some point the saying "stress makes you fat" – well in this case there is quite a body of evidence behind it. This is not just stress from cardio but also from other areas of life such as work, family, relationships, friends, money etc. All of these factors increase cortisol levels and this can prohibit weight loss. Exercise physiologist and nutritional biochemist Shaun Talbott has researched this and found that high cortisol levels not only make it difficult to lose weight but can also weaken the immune system and contribute towards hypertension, diabetes, depression and osteoporosis[3]. The easiest way to combat this if you have tried and not really managed to eradicate stress is to reach for the Chinese herbs as there are many available that reduce stress without making you drowsy. One great example that I take is a combination of Rehmannia and Schizandra. Other well documented herbs that do a similar thing include Ashwaghanda, Holy basil, Siberian Ginseng and Rhodiola. A trip to my local health food store was all it took for my stresses to evaporate and the fact that it's a kind of training aid by reducing the hormone that can make you fat is a perfect benefit. Bring herbs into your life and you won't be sorry.

Cardio Junkies and skinny fat

I can sense that there may be panic over the cardio comments so now let's just tackle this in parts. First of all I am not advocating that you cut all cardio out of your routine – because done well and done in moderation it will assist in you achieving your dream physique (a 10k run at race pace can burn up to 800 calories). Similarly any cardio is better than just sitting on the sofa at home! Cardio needs to be present but should not necessarily be considered as the main part of your fitness regime – that spot needs to be wisely reserved for weight training.

I myself was the worst case of a "cardio junkie" – running for LPS Athletics requires high mileage training on the track and on the road. For the last three years I have been running anywhere between 50-70 miles a week. No wonder I had developed muscle wastage across my back, had a painful winging scapula and wondered why I would get injured anytime I lifted anything around the house! Many people in life are stuck in similar scenarios - they are "skinny-fat" in the way that they have poor muscular structure and a high fat storage, yet on the outside they look fairly ok - despite this internal imbalance of muscle to fat. This is due to inadequate training with weights. Those days are long gone for me, I realise during cross country season I need to incorporate longer runs into my schedule, but it's not at the expense of my resistance and circuit weights sessions, it's all about finding that perfect balance which for me works easily in Spring and Summer, when I can co-ordinate weights sessions with sprint intervals at the track; it all works well at developing power, strength and speed.

This gets a little harder in the winter when running longer mileage, but this builds up endurance which helps in longer circuits and as long as I keep my protein intake up and fit in weights sessions during the week, it seems to be the winning combination for me. Some people need to do lots of cardio as it makes them feel better and makes them feel like they have had a good workout, but remember if you are one of those people, doing too much cardio can prohibit the sculpting of muscles and body tone. Find your balance and then keep it there to realise your dream physique.

Making cardio routines more effective – Interval training

Before we move on to the subject of weights we need to stick on cardio to explore what types of cardio are effective to incorporate into your fitness regime. The key to getting real results from your cardio is all about introducing intervals.

Without any change or peaks and troughs in the workout you hit a plateau, the body adapts – it finds a comfortable patch to work in and so then you don't see any results! Researchers at the University of Copenhagen found that Interval training improves cardiorespiratory fitness and glucose tolerance[4]. By introducing intervals to your cardio, you are effectively asking the body to respond to a shock and a challenge and it will feel good. It will be achievable as you will have a short recovery time after each interval. See below for suggested HIIT (High intensity interval training) regimes:

Cardio Sessions to pick from - all 20 mins max	Warm up	Effort on resistance	Recover	Repeat	Comments
Bike, X Trainer, Runner, Rower	2 mins	1 min	1 min	x 9 times	Good one to start on
Bike, X Trainer, Runner, Rower	2 mins	2 mins	1 min	x 6 times	Recovery getting shorter so you need energy for this
Bike, X Trainer, Runner, Rower	2 mins	1 min	30 secs	x 12 times	Hard and fast interval session
Bike, X Trainer, Runner, Rower	2 mins	2 mins	30 secs	x 7 times	Good one to feel the burn
Bike, X Trainer, Runner, Rower	2 mins	18 mins tempo	None	Only do once	Hard to maintain the pace but it needs to be at tempo otherwise you will just float along too easily

The good news is that these interval sessions only last about 20 minutes and they may well be more beneficial for you than the 40 or 60 minutes you would normally spend or would potentially plan to spend on cardio. Think fast and frenetic. Think effort and strength. This will cut down the amount of time you spend working out or hitting the gym for sure. This was one of the best things for me as I used to lose a lot of time during the day in the gym, now my time in there is shorter and I am getting totally and dramatically different results all for the better.

Interval training is naturally harder as it requires effort but that's the key, the higher the effort, the better the results you will see. You can also play around with these cardio intervals and remember to keep changing it – the more you change your routines, the less chance your body has to adapt so that you will continue to see good results from those changes. Steady state cardio can still be thrown in to your weekly schedule in moderation to help recovery in those interval sessions as it builds endurance but once a week is fine, twice is more than enough. Anymore and that's where your hard work on physique building will be lost and you will be frustrated by not getting anywhere.

Tabata

One of the best and shortest workouts for a ridiculously high energy cardiovascular burst is that of Tabata. Created by Izumi Tabata, it has often been referred to as the world's greatest fat burning workout and works on the premise that the higher the exercise intensity the higher the proportion of fat loss as it really boosts overall metabolism. There are a lot of other similar techniques that Tabata has sparked off but the original protocol is based on 20 seconds of effort (repetitions) followed by 10 seconds rest and this is repeated for 8 cycles. The whole session would last 4 minutes or 240 seconds which you may laugh at on initial thought, but the likelihood is you will be on the floor after that 4 minutes and it will feel like you have worked out for an hour! You would select a specific exercise such as a squat, lunge, press up or sit up and put that into the regime of those 8 cycles. Other variations could be practised on a cardio machine or with weights or a number of cardio machines or weights to turn it into a circuit. Weighted exercises would be my choice for a Tabata session as it conditions the body and you will burn more body fat afterwards in comparison to a longer cardio session[5]. Have a think about when you could fit this into your week, it's easy to find 4 minutes (or 8 minutes if you think you are hard enough to tackle two sessions at a time), but this would only be needed a couple of times a week in addition to your regular workouts. It is also recommended that you don't try and fit in any other really tough exercise on the day you do this, as you will be feeling pretty tired and your body will probably need the rest – especially if you build your Tabata session up in to mini circuits.

Time to lift weights – it's the best way to reduce body fat!

On to the world of weights and before you winch and think of images of beefy body builders, I have to stop you right there! It is one of the most ridiculous of myths that lifting weights will make you big and bulky. It is actually the reverse as when you lift the weights and you are controlling the weight and keeping tension on the muscle you are actually sculpting the body and so making yourself look more defined, more toned and more athletic. Yes you may weigh a little more (as muscle weighs more than fat) but if you look leaner then surely that is the result, so just throw out those scales! You need to let go of any hang ups regarding a particular weight you want to get to, instead just use the mirror and a measure tape as an indication of how you are looking. The same principle applies to clothing sizes – unless you shoot up a group of sizes, there is no need to get too hung up on what you are wearing as long as it looks good on you and makes you feel good that is all that matters. Researchers at the University of Turku in Finland found that weight training builds bone density, improves muscle mass, decreases fat mass, burns abdominal fat, reduces blood pressure, enhances insulin sensitivity and improves glucose tolerance[6]. The findings even state that it should be a central component of any public health campaign! Lifting weights will be the best thing you can do to help reduce your body fat, not running around park after park after park! When I was running six days a week and not putting any effort into weights, my body fat remained exactly the same for 3 years. Then I started to enter the world of weights and here is what happened to my body fat percentages (with a little help from Poliquin supplements covered in Chapter 3):

Feb	15th	2011	26.9%	(This is where I had been for 3+ years)
April	20th	2011	19.9%	
June	11th	2011	17.9%	
Aug	22nd	2011	17.7%	
Nov	18th	2011	15.8%	
June	8th	2012	14.9%	
Nov	9th	2012	13.1%	

Poliquin™ BioSignature Modulation Results

This is coming down all the time as I continue to train with weights 3+ times a week.

Now we all have to start somewhere in the game of weights and I remember lifting 4kg weights and thinking I would never be able to increase that 4kg ever! Now I always grin at that weight as I reach for the 10kg dumbbell. Now take a look at the picture on the next page and try to spot the bulk on me! It is not there and never will be because I am not ingesting any natural or unnatural supplementation to make me bulky and I am not working out in a way that would make me look like the hulk!

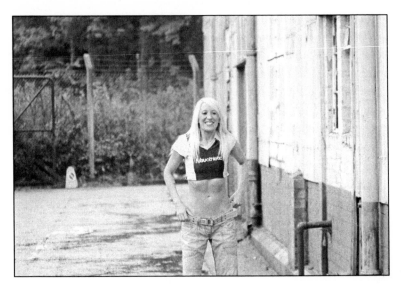

No bulk but a new belt is needed to keep my jeans up!

Technique & Progression

When you start lifting weights, the key is to home in on the right technique, not to rush the movement and to keep an amount of tension to really work the muscle. As you continue to do this you will make small increases in weight each week which will also be partly as a result of your diet, your supplementation and your state of mind covered in the next three chapters. Even the smallest of increases should be applauded because if you keep adding weights in small amounts, before you know it you will have travelled quite a distance from your original starting weight. It's really important to remember that the more muscle the body has, the more calories it uses even when resting so increasing your muscle mass will assist in overall weight loss i.e. loss of fat not muscle. That's exactly what happened to me in just over a year or so.

Main methods of weight training

Now on to the types of weight training. You have a number of options and the most popular types used for their effectiveness are as follows:

1. Multiple sets and reps of the same exercise e.g. 10 reps of Bicep curls × 3 sets
2. Supersets – this refers to two sets of different exercises performed with little or no rest back to back e.g. Bicep curl 10 reps + Tricep kickback 10 reps × 3 sets
3. Pyramid Sets – here you would start with light weights and perform a high number of reps, then you would finish on heavier weights but perform fewer reps. e.g. 1. Chest press 24 reps with 20kg barbell; 2. Chest press 12 reps 30kg; 3. Chest press 6 reps 40kg. (This can also be practised with different exercises for an all over body blast). The weights mentioned here are just examples, so modify this to work for your strength.
4. Drop Sets – This refers to the method of training where you would start with heavy weights on a low number of reps and finish on lighter weights performing a greater amount of reps, so the opposite to Pyramid Sets. e.g Lat pull down 50kg × 6 reps; Lat pull down 40kg × 12 reps; Lat pull down 30kg × 24 reps (again this could be done on different exercises instead of this isolation example).

A basic theme follows through all weighted exercises and that is if you want to burn fat, think light to moderate weights at a fairly swift tempo with a high number of reps which turns into a good cardiovascular workout. If you want to build more muscle, think heavier weights at a slow controlled tempo for only a small number of reps to build strength.

The importance of change

As with cardio, it only takes a matter of time before your body adapts to the weights program you are practising so they need to be kept fresh. Here are some of the general rules I follow before we look at the actual different programs:

- If it's a fat burning weights circuit, I will only practice 2 × per week for a max of 4 weeks before changing the circuit.
- If it's an isolation weights session per muscle group, I will do this for anywhere between 4-6 weeks before changing.
- If it's an upper body-lower body mix, I will practice this 2 × per week and complete for 3-4 weeks.
- If it is a drop set session per muscle group (going from 6 to 12 to 24 reps on an exercise), I will usually practise for 4 weeks. Same principle for pyramid training.
- Every 2-3 months I will take a whole week off lifting any weights.
- I make sure I have at least one complete rest day per week. Rest is very important and will allow your body to repair and grow to its full potential.

> "Periodisation is very important,
> 3 × 4 week phases in a 12 week cycle
> is a winning formula"
> J. Slomka, Primal Health

Taking all this into account, on the next few pages there is a program that you can follow for up to 16 weeks then go back to the start and follow again for roughly three times with a couple of weeks rest thrown in to cover your next full year's workout plan! I have added weeks 13-16 as an optional month for those who prefer to do a few different things before returning back to the start after a 12 week cycle. If you prefer you can still train in 3x4 week cycles going back to the start every 12 weeks. This would mean that you would do the entire 12 week program 4 times a year (with a couple of weeks rest thrown in). For those wanting to add another month on to this, you simply follow the complete 4x4 week cycle going back to the start every 16 weeks. Both options have been mentioned to suit the time constraints currently in your life. No matter which one you choose to follow, by the time you get back to the start your body will have forgotten the effects of each workout plan, so you will be able to get results and continue to make improvements in muscle tone, definition and overall fitness. I personally prefer the 16 week cycle method because it all seems slightly less familiar when you return to week 1! So you now have a perpetual training calendar you can take to the gym each time you train. To make life easier, all exercises mentioned in the fitness plans are available to view online at www.gonein60minutes. co.uk so you can identify any you don't recognise or just generally check your technique is right.

Rest and Rehab!

It's just as important to give your body the right amount of rest as it is to make sure you work it out properly, yet it's an area many overlook. Aim to have at least one or two days off a week to rest and recover. Listen to your body, if something aches to the point of being too painful to train with, then rest and return to the workouts when you recover. If you pick up any injuries in sports, fitness or any other areas of life, take time to treat them and really consider the physiotherapy options available to you.

I have found ultrasound good for breaking up any scar tissues and reducing inflammation on minor niggles but for some of my longer term injuries I have found Active Release Techniques (ART®) the most effective. Don't be surprised if you have not heard about this, it's one of those best kept secrets in the world of physiotherapy and is used by many top athletes and performers in America. It is growing in popularity in the UK and is definitely worth investigating if you feel that a particular injury is holding you back. It's also good for improving general flexibility. In a study conducted on 20 healthy males, it was found that ART greatly improved hamstring flexibility by an average of 8.3cm and the effects were felt immediately after treatment[7]. Search on www.activerelease.com for your nearest practitioner.

Sleep

Although sleep is not an exercise, I want you to think about it in on two dimensions – firstly enough sleep will make sure that you operate at your optimum level in your gym sessions and daily workouts. Secondly sleep is the time where stresses should dissolve themselves and cortisol levels should be nice and low – so think of sleep as an extra dimension that will assist in your quest to achieve your dream body. Countless studies have shown that people who have enough sleep and of a good quality are often the slimmest and trimmest of people. Dr Shahrad Taheri, a consultant endocrinologist at Birmingham Heartlands Hospital, found that people who sleep for less than 4 hours a night are 73% more likely to gain excess weight and eat more throughout the day[8]. Lack of sleep has also been linked to high levels of cortisol and a variety of age-related diseases[9] .During your sleep the body releases growth hormone which is essential for maintaining a healthy immune system, tissue repair and body fat reduction, so get counting those z's as soon as you can! I always aim for a minimum of 8 hours which most cite as the perfect amount of time to rest for. Last point on sleep – if you have trouble getting a good night's sleep;

take one or two magnesium tablets one hour before bed and problem solved.

> "Lack of magnesium is a barrier to sleep. Eliminate this sleep barrier by supplementing with Magnesium"
> J. Slomka, Primal Health

Summary

- Reduce the long sessions of flat cardio (1 or 2 times a week is plenty) and replace your other cardio sessions with interval training.
- Pick up the weights, they will not make you bulky but they will send your metabolic rate racing.
- Consider taking Chinese herbs to reduce stress and cortisol levels.
- Practise the Tabata method – it's only a few minutes once or twice a week and it's great for body conditioning.
- Make small increases in weight each week for best effects as the body will adapt, so don't get into a comfortable way of training – make every rep matter.
- Vary your weights workouts – you can chose from multiple sets, supersets, pyramid sets or drop sets.
- Listen to your body, take rest when you need it and don't ignore any injuries – get them treated and move on!
- Make sure you aim for a minimum of 8 hours sleep to keep your body in top condition.

Weeks 1-4: Overview

DAY	CARDIO	WEIGHTS SESSION	ABS
Mon	Body Fat Blitz Circuit 45 mins	*No isolated body parts in wks 1-4*	*None in wks 1-4*
Tue			
Wed	Body Fat Blitz Circuit 45 mins		
Thu			
Fri	Tabata Circuit 20 mins		
Sat			
Sun			

Weeks 1-4:

- The aim is to blitz fat before building muscle and requires you to work out 3 DAYS PER WEEK - of your choice.
- Compound circuits are for all over body tone and they double up as cardiovascular workouts - read on for more details on these workouts.
- Tabata circuit is only 20 mins but will awaken the heart and feel like the hardest workout you have ever done.
- After week 4 the body is ready to start working on isolated muscle groups.
- This first 4 week period will reduce body fat % considerably.
- Cardio is introduced from week 5 where breathing will be ready for interval sessions.
- Read on for full breakdowns of all workouts during weeks 1-4.

Weeks 5-8: Overview

DAY	CARDIO	WEIGHTS SESSION BODY PART	ABS
Mon		Chest & Back ("6,12,25")	Abs (A)
Tue	Tabata circuit 20 mins		
Wed		Legs ("6,12,25")	
Thu			
Fri	20 mins interval on bike/x train/runner	Bicep and Tricep ("6,12,25")	Abs (B)
Sat			
Sun			

Weeks 5-8:

- This requires you to work out 4 DAYS PER WEEK - on days of your choice but you will not be in the gym more than 40 mins max at any point!
- Tabata workout is to be done on different days to your isolated body parts weight session.
- Isolated body parts will work on your body tone and will start to "cut" muscles.
- Read on for full breakdowns of all workouts during weeks 5-8.

Weeks 9-12: Overview

DAY	CARDIO	WEIGHTS SESSION BODY PART	ABS
Mon	Body Fat Blitz Circuit 45 mins		
Tue		Back (wks 11,12)	
Wed	20 min interval cardio runner/x train/bike	Legs (wks 11,12)	
Thu			
Fri	Body Conditioning 20 mins	Bicep and Tricep (wks 11,12)	
Sat			
Sun			

Weeks 9-12:

- The fat blitz circuit at this phase will be different to the one you practised in weeks 1-4 for maximum effect.
- You will rest muscle groups for weeks 9 and 10.
- Weeks 11 and 12 you will drop one circuit (either body conditioning or fat blitz) and do 2 weeks on the weights isolation program again.
- You will be working out for between 3-4 DAYS PER WEEK.
- Isolated muscle groups will start to really carve definition.
- Read on for full breakdowns of all workouts during weeks 9-12.

Weeks 13-16: Overview

DAY	CARDIO	WEIGHTS SESSION BODY PART	ABS
Mon	Cardio interval x 20 min runner/x train/bike	Upper Body Weights	
Tue		Lower Body Weights	Abs (A)
Wed			
Thu	Cardio interval x 20 min runner/x train/bike	Upper Body Weights	
Fri		Lower Body Weights	Abs (B)
Sat			
Sun			

Weeks 13-16:

- Breaks upper and lower body workouts apart and builds tone.
- This requires you to work out 4 DAYS PER WEEK.
- Cardio can be chosen on either of the upper or lower body workout days.
- Abs can also be done on either day. Combining it with legs will be effective as Abs are already worked well on the legs program.
- Read on for full breakdowns of all workouts during weeks 13-16.

Weeks 1-4: Complete Programs

Muscle Group:	All over body fat blitz
Program Timing:	Wks 1-4
Warm up:	5 Mins cardio - any discipline
Active Stretches performed at start:	Squats, push ups, lunges, arm swings and circles (no weights for this).
Static Stretches performed at end:	Hip flexors, quads, hamstrings, calves and glutes (holding for 30 seconds).
Notes on how to perform circuit:	Do all the A's x 3 before moving onto the B's - each letter represents a circuit.

EXERCISE	SETS	REPS	REST	WEIGHT (make a note each wk in this box)
A1 - Russian step ups with dumbbells	3	15	10 secs	
A2 - Barbell deadlifts	3	15	10 secs	
A3 - Calf raises with dumbbell	3	15	90 secs	
B1 - Wide grip pulldown on machine	3	15	10 secs	
B2 - Push press with dumbbells	3	15	20 secs	
B3 - Dumbbell bent row	3	15	60 secs	
C1 - Dumbbell hammer curls	3	15	10 secs	
C2 - Dumbbell tricep extensions	3	15	10 secs	
C3 - Jacknife swiss ball	3	15	75 secs	
D1 - Squat push press with dumbbells	8	8	30 secs	

Muscle Group:

Program Timing:

Warm up:

Active Stretches performed at start:

Static Stretches performed at end:

Notes on how to perform cicruit:

All over Tabata session

Wks 1-4

5 Mins cardio - any discipline

Squats, push ups, lunges, arm swings and circles (no weights for this).

Hip flexors, quads, hamstrings, calves and glutes (holding for 30 seconds).

20 seconds on, 10 seconds off x 4 times for each exercise, 1 min rest between exercises 1-5. Do this circuit a total of 2 times for each tabata session.

EXERCISE	SETS	REPS	REST	WEIGHT (make a note each wk in this box)
1. Kettlebell swings	20 secs	2	1 min	
2. Reverse lunge with dumbbells	20 secs	2	1 min	
3. Persian press ups - bodyweight only	20 secs	2	1 min	
4. Squat jumps with dumbbells or bodyweight	20 secs	2	1 min	
5. Russian twist on swiss ball with one dumbell to twist with	20 secs	2	1 min	

Weeks 5-8: Complete Programs

Muscle Group: Chest & Back
Program Timing: Wks 5-8
Warm up: 5 Mins cardio - any discipline
Active Stretches performed at start: Squats, push ups, lunges, arm swings and circles (no weights for this).
Static Stretches performed at end: Hip flexors, quads, hamstrings, calves and glutes (holding for 30 seconds).
Notes on how to perform circuit: Do all the A's x 3 before moving onto the B's - each letter represents a circuit. Decrease the weights as the reps increase.

EXERCISE	SETS	REPS	REST	WEIGHT (make a note each wk in this box)
Chest				
A1 - Incline dumbbell press	3	6	15 secs	(Heavy)
A2 - Incline barbell press	3	12	15 secs	(Moderate)
A3 - Low incline dumbbell press	3	25	2 mins	(Lighter)
Back				
B1 - Chin ups (assisted for beginners)	3	6	15 secs	(Heavy)
B2 - Dumbbell bent row	3	12	15 secs	(Moderate)
B3 - Cable row to neck on machine	3	25	2 mins	(Lighter)

Muscle Group: Triceps & Biceps

Program Timing: Wks 5-8

Warm up: 5 Mins cardio - any discipline

Active Stretches performed at start: Squats, push ups, lunges, arm swings and circles (no weights for this).

Static Stretches performed at end: Hip flexors, quads, hamstrings, calves and glutes (holding for 30 seconds).

Notes on how to perform cicruit: Do all the A's x 3 before moving onto the B's - each letter represents a circuit. Decrease the weights as the reps increase.

EXERCISE	SETS	REPS	REST	WEIGHT (make a note each wk in this box)
Triceps				
A1 - Dips (optional to use weight between ankles)	3	6	15 secs	(Heavy)
A2 - Decline barbell extensions	3	12	15 secs	(Moderate)
A3 - Cable press downs on machine	3	25	2 mins	(Lighter)
Biceps				
B1 - Incline dumbbell curls	3	6	15 secs	(Heavy)
B2 - Dumbbell hammer curls	3	12	15 secs	(Moderate)
B3 - Barbell curls	3	25	2 mins	(Lighter)

Muscle Group: Legs
Program Timing: Wks 5-8
Warm up: 5 Mins cardio - any discipline
Active Stretches performed at start: Squats, push ups, lunges, arm swings and circles (no weights for this).
Static Stretches performed at end: Hip flexors, quads, hamstrings, calves and glutes (holding for 30 seconds).
Notes on how to perform cicruit: Do all the A's x 3 before moving onto the B's - each letter represents a circuit.
Decrease the weights as the reps increase.

EXERCISE	SETS	REPS	REST	WEIGHT (make a note each wk in this box)
Quads				
A1 - Dumbbell squats	3	6	15 secs	(Heavy)
A2 - Alternating lunges with dumbbbells	3	12	15 secs	(Moderate)
A3 - Leg extensions on machine	3	25	2 mins	(Lighter)
Hamstrings				
B1 - Leg curls on machine	3	6	15 secs	(Heavy)
B2 - Romanian Deadlifts with barbell	3	12	15 secs	(Moderate)
B3 - Back extensions on swiss ball or machine	3	25	2 mins	(Lighter)

Muscle Group: Abs

Program Timing: Wks 5-8 (Workout A)

Warm up: 5 Mins cardio - any discipline

Active Stretches performed at start: Squats, push ups, lunges, arm swings and circles (no weights for this).

Static Stretches performed at end: Hip flexors, quads, hamstrings, calves and glutes (holding for 30 seconds).

Notes on how to perform cicruit: Work through all 7 excercises once then repeat them all x 3 so you will have completed 4 sets to finish.

EXERCISE	SETS	REPS	REST	WEIGHT (make a note each wk in this box)
A1 - Hanging garhammer raises - bodyweight	4	20	0	
A2 - Weighted crunches on swiss ball with a dumbell/disc	4	10	0	
A3 - Dumbbell roll outs	4	10	0	
A4 - Jacknife Swiss ball	4	10	0	
A5 - Dumbbell russian twist (seated on floor)	4	15 p/side	0	
A6 - Leg raises (together) - bodyweight or small ankle weights	4	15	0	
A7 - Plank on swiss ball - bodyweight	4	Max hold	90 secs	

Muscle Group: Abs
Program Timing: Wks 5-8 (Workout B)
Warm up: 5 Mins cardio - any discipline
Active Stretches performed at start: Squats, push ups, lunges, arm swings and circles (no weights for this).
Static Stretches performed at end: Hip flexors, quads, hamstrings, calves and glutes (holding for 30 seconds).
Notes on how to perform cicruit: Do all the A's before moving onto the B's etc - each letter represents a circuit.

EXERCISE	SETS	REPS	REST	WEIGHT (make a note each wk in this box)
A1 - Spiderman push ups - bodyweight	4	10-12	10 secs	
A2 - Side plank lateral raise with dumbbell	4	6 p/side	10 secs	
A3 - Cross body mountain climbers - bodyweight	4	10 p/leg	10 secs	
A4 - Floor wipers with barbell	4	10 p/side	10 secs	
A5 - Dumbbell roll outs	4	10	60 secs	

Weeks 9-12: Complete Programs

Muscle Group: All over body fat blitz

Program Timing: Wks 9-12

Warm up: 5 Mins cardio - any discipline

Active Stretches perfomed at start: Squats, push ups, lunges, arm swings and circles (no weights for this).

Static Stretches performed at end: Hip flexors, quads, hamstrings, calves and glutes (holding for 30 seconds).

Notes on how to perform circuit: Do all the A's x 3 before moving onto the B's etc - each letter represents a circuit.

EXERCISE	SETS	REPS	REST	WEIGHT (make a note each wk in this box)
A1 - Squat push press with dumbbells	3	10-12	0	
A2 - Reverse lunge with dumbbells	3	20	30 secs	
B1 - Squat curl with dumbbells	3	10-12	0	
B2 - Spiderman push-ups - bodyweight only	3	8-10	30 secs	
C1 - Lunge rotation with dumbbells	3	20	0	
C2 - Renegade row with dumbbells	3	8-10	30 secs	
D1 - Lunge to overhead with dumbbells	2	20	0	
D2 - Single leg swiss ball curls - bodyweight only	2	20	30 secs	

Muscle Group: All over body conditioning
Program Timing: Wks 9-12
Warm up: 5 Mins cardio - any discipline
Active Stretches performed at start: Squats, push ups, lunges, arm swings and circles (no weights for this).
Static Stretches performed at end: Hip flexors, quads, hamstrings, calves and glutes (holding for 30 seconds).
Notes on how to perform circuit: 30 seconds on, 30 seconds off x 8 (6 for last two) times for each exercise, 30 seconds rest between exercises 1-5. Do this circuit only once a week for a conditioning session.

EXERCISE	SETS	REPS	REST	WEIGHT (make a note each wk in this box)
1. Squat-curl-press with dumbbells	8	1	30 secs	
2. Chin ups - bodyweight or small weight between ankles	8	1	30 secs	
3. Kettlebell swings	8	1	30 secs	
4. Walking lunges with dumbbells	6	1	30 secs	
5. Persian press ups with twist	6	1	30 secs	

Weeks 13-16: Complete Programs

Muscle Group: Upper body accumulation
Program Timing: Wks 13-16
Warm up: 5 Mins cardio - any discipline
Active Stretches perfomed at start: Squats, push ups, lunges, arm swings and circles (no weights for this).
Static Stretches performed at end: Hip flexors, quads, hamstrings, calfs and glutes (holding for 30 seconds).
Notes on how to perform cicruit: Do all the A's before moving onto the B's etc - each letter represents a circuit. Increase sets each week then deload for last week.

EXERCISE	SETS	REPS	REST	WEIGHT (make a note each wk in this box)
A1 - Chest press machine	3(wk1), 4 (wk2), 5 (wk3), 3 (wk4)	10-12	20 secs	
A2 - Chin ups (assisted for beginners)	3(wk1), 4 (wk2), 5 (wk3), 3 (wk4)	8-10	60 secs	
B1 - Shoulder press machine	3(wk1), 4 (wk2), 5 (wk3), 3 (wk4)	10-12	20 secs	
B2 - Single arm dumbbell row	3(wk1), 4 (wk2), 5 (wk3), 3 (wk4)	8-10	60 secs	
C1 - Dips - bodyweight only	3(wk1), 4 (wk2), 5 (wk3), 3 (wk4)	8-10	20 secs	
C2 - Kneeling Zottman curl with dumbbells	3(wk1), 4 (wk2), 5 (wk3), 3 (wk4)	10-12	60 secs	

Muscle Group: Lower body accumulation

Program Timing: Wks 13-16

Warm up: 5 Mins cardio - any discipline

Active Stretches performed at start: Squats, push ups, lunges, arm swings and circles (no weights for this).

Static Stretches performed at end: Hip flexors, quads, hamstrings, calfs and glutes (holding for 30 seconds).

Notes on how to perform cricuit: Do all the A's before moving onto the B's etc - each letter represents a circuit. Increase sets each week then deload for last week.

EXERCISE	SETS	REPS	REST	WEIGHT (make a note each wk in this box)
A1 - Dumbbell split squats	3(wk1), 4 (wk2), 5 (wk3), 3 (wk4)	10-12	30 secs	
A2 - Swiss ball curl (feet inward) - bodyweight	3(wk1), 4 (wk2), 5 (wk3), 3 (wk4)	15-20	60 secs	
B1 - Dumbbell step ups	3(wk1), 4 (wk2), 5 (wk3), 3 (wk4)	10-12	30 secs	
B2 - Barbell deadlifts	3(wk1), 4 (wk2), 5 (wk3), 3 (wk4)	10-12	60 secs	
C1 - Calf raises with dumbbells	3(wk1), 4 (wk2), 5 (wk3), 3 (wk4)	15	30 secs	
C2 - Abs crunch on machine	3(wk1), 4 (wk2), 5 (wk3), 3 (wk4)	10-12	60 secs	

Muscle Group: Abs (Workout A)

Program Timing: **Wks 13-16**

Warm up: 5 Mins cardio - any discipline

Active Stretches performed at start: Squats, push ups, lunges, arm swings and circles (no weights for this).

Static Stretches performed at end: Hip flexors, quads, hamstrings, calves and glutes (holding for 30 seconds).

Notes on how to perform circuit: Do all the A's before moving onto the B's etc - each letter represents a circuit.

EXERCISE	SETS	REPS	REST	WEIGHT (make a note each wk in this box)
A1 - Traditional crunch with weight above chest	4	20		
A2 - Hip thrusts (legs straight) - bodyweight	4	20		
A3 - Oblique crunches - bodyweight	4	10 each side		
A4 - Jacknife swiss ball	4	15		
A5 - V-sit ups - bodyweight	4	10		

Muscle Group: Abs (Workout B)

Program Timing: Wks 13-16

Warm up: 5 Mins cardio - any discipline

Active Stretches performed at start: Squats, push ups, lunges, arm swings and circles (no weights for this).

Static Stretches performed at end: Hip flexors, quads, hamstrings, calves and glutes (holding for 30 seconds).

Notes on how to perform circuit: Do all the A's before moving onto the B's etc - each letter represents a circuit.

EXERCISE	SETS	REPS	REST	WEIGHT (make a note each wk in this box)
A1 - Hanging garhammer raises -bodyweight	4	20		
A2 - Butterfly kicks - bodyweight	4	20		
A3 - Dumbbell russian twist (seated on floor)	4	15		
A4 - Single knee crunch - bodyweight	4	10 each leg		
A5 - Long lever crunches (dumbbells over head, arms straight)	4	15		

CHAPTER 2 - DIET

Green eating for greater gains

We may as well start on another controversial point after digesting the last chapter's crusade for weight lifting techniques! You are now going to be introduced to clean eating for a better life – it starts with V and ends in egan! Before you laugh, dismiss this and move on to the next part, let's start by having a look at some superstar athletes who have all opted for the Vegan diet:

Famous Vegan Athletes
Carl Lewis - Multi Olympic gold medallist for 100m, 200m, long jump & 100m relays
Jane Black – Female weightlifting champion
Molly Cameron – Female bike racing champion
Mac Danzig - Male mixed martial arts champion
Tony Gonzalez - 6' 5", 246 lb. Male NFL tight end for the Atlanta Falcons
Keith Holmes - Male middleweight boxing champion
Scott Jurek - Two-time Male winner of the Badwater Ultramarathon
Billie Jean King - Female tennis champion
Martina Navratilova - Female tennis champion
Pat Neshek - 6' 3", 210 lb. Male pitcher for the Minnesota Twins
Fiona Oakes - Female cyclist and record-breaking marathon champion
Bill Pearl - Four-time Mr. Universe winner
Pat Reeves - Female marathon runner turned bodybuilding champion
Weia Reinbound – Female world record holder in high-jumping
James Southwood - Male kickboxing champion
Ed Templeton - Male professional skateboarding champion
Kenneth Williams - America's first male vegan bodybuilding champion
Martyn Moxon - Male English cricketer who played ten yests and eight one day internationals for England

Now that is some collection of super athletic and successful people.

But aren't all Vegans weak?

Now let's blow the myth that Vegans are weak, skinny and have no strength by looking at Scott Jurek. Scott completed the Badwater Ultramarathon which is thought to be the toughest extreme-sport marathon on earth. You battle with 115-degree heat, moving for 135 nonstop miles all the way from Death Valley to Mount Whitney. Just to put that in perspective that's running just over five normal marathons all in one go – more than impressive I say! Surely you don't win that many Gold medals like the legendary Carl Lewis if you are so weak! Maybe it's time to realise the powers of plant protein and watch your body change as you do this – give it a try, what have you got to lose other than weight! Plant proteins are lower in fat and cholesterol in comparison to animal proteins and they are often higher in fibre, micronutirents and lower in calories. They are low in Vitamin B12 but that can easily be purchased in way of a supplement from your local health food store.

It's a moral thing

It's obvious that there are many successful sportsmen and athletes that practice veganism and it does not hold them back from achieving and there are hundreds more athletes at various levels doing the same thing that I have not mentioned here. Aside from the fact that many of these athletes believe that plant based proteins are healthier for you, many share my belief that you should not rely on animals for any ingredients be it their bodies, their skin or their fats. I adore animals more so than humans in most cases and I just could not morally bring myself to do it. I even have a tattoo on my arm with a huge V for Vegan with the words cruelty free underneath it and various animal footprints on my inside bicep (I am not advocating you go out and get a tattoo but it shows the extent of my cause). There are healthier, cleaner and cruelty free options to follow and you get that with a green diet. Now I am not naive enough to believe that everyone is going to be converted to the world of veganism after reading this book, but you are at least in possession of some very interesting information here that shows you that success and veganism seem to run along the same path.

If you are committed to giving this a try for a week, a month, a year or a lifetime, read the book "Skinny Bitch" as it will very bluntly deliver all the info to you on the contamination levels in meats, fish and dairy as well as giving you an insight to how much abuse the animals in those industries are subject to. I have been Vegetarian since the age of 6 and turned Vegan at 24. Most people start off as Vegetarians as it's quite a change from meat eater straight to Vegan and so Vegetarian for me was the middle ground until there were enough alternatives and substitutes on the market which is definitely now the case. Paul McCartney's "Meat free Mondays" have taken off really well now across the globe and have started to make people really consider their diets and more importantly the effect of those diets on their long term health. Why not start there, give it a try and see how you feel. I have more energy than anyone I know, I never get any colds, I am really wired for life and everyone who meets me always say the same thing – that they are surprised to find out I am a Vegan (not a Vulcan as quite a few people have joked!).

For those who just can't take the jump and feel they need meat, fish and dairy, your choices will also be covered in this chapter so don't worry, I am not that cruel!

The importance of protein

Ok so let's get to the most important diet advice. If you want to drop those extra pounds of fat and tone up your body then you need to consider your protein sources as your new best friends. There has been so much said on the subject of protein – many in the past have followed the Atkins Diet and reported positive results and the majority of body conscious people you meet these days are trying to minimise carbs and maximise proteins and all for good reasons. Protein not only makes you look trimmer in the long run but it also reduces those hunger cravings so you don't have to go down the route of appetite suppressants if you manage this part of your diet correctly. So where can you get your protein from?

Main Meals

If you are not veggie/vegan you will be aware that meat, fish and dairy contain high levels of protein so think steak, think chicken salads, tuna, eggs etc. If you are vegetarian you have quorn and some of the meat alternative brands such as Linda McCartney. If you are vegan you have tofu, gardein, tempeh and seiten as your main options - most of which can be bought at your local health food store. To accompany these you have the options of beans, pulses and legumes which are all super rich in protein. Add some nutritious vegetables and that's a perfect meal sorted (this does not include chips!).

Snacks

Smaller portions of the above, peanut butter, nuts, seeds, protein bars.

Shakes/Bars

Whey protein for those meat eaters or veggies. Soya, pea, rice or hemp protein for vegans.

> "Protein stimulates
> neurotransmitters in the brain to
> wake up the nervous system, so it's
> good to eat protein at breakfast"
> J. Slomka, Primal Health

For those who run and worry that high protein diets are not suitable… think again. In her book "Secrets from America's top female runner", Suzy Favor Hamilton talks openly about the fact that low fat diets harm runners and they need to understand the importance of protein in order to recover from any muscle soreness and that the benefits of a high protein diet far outweigh the risks[10].

So exactly how much protein do you need during the day? The general RDA for protein intake is 56g for men and 46g for women. According to Donald Layman Ph.D – a professor at the University of Illinois, this is too low and you should aim for 1.5g of protein for every kg of bodyweight[11]. Layman also stresses that this kind of diet can still be effective for weight loss even on restricted exercise days by stabilising blood glucose, increasing the loss of body fat and reducing the loss of lean muscle. I aim to get over the 100g mark where possible on weight training days as directed by my Personal Trainer who advocates 2g of protein per kilogram body weight. This follows the same guidelines as set by the international society of sports nutrition who state between 1.4-2.0g per kg of bodyweight for weight training[12].

What about carbohydrates?

Carbs contain water which is retained in the muscles making you look fuller and often in many cases bloated! Out of total curiosity, I completed a 6 month diet based on consuming very little carbs, eating them only for my breakfast in porridge and having carb gels around my training sessions and I honestly felt as though I had lost a layer around my whole body. The first week or so I really struggled for energy as I was used to overloading on cereals, pasta, rice and bread but my body soon adapted. Now I am not advocating that you completely cut out carbs altogether, as they are the main source of energy in daily diets but choose complex, good carbs (wholemeal, wholegrain, bran, barley, oats, buckwheat, fruit and vegetables). Steer clear from white or bleached foods; think natural and often in most cases, think brown i.e. swap white rice for brown, swap white bread for brown etc.

Eating the right things at the right time

It's really important to combine these food groups around training sessions too; you can't go wrong if you choose the heavier carbs as your pre-workout foods to provide endurance, strength and high energy. They top up your energy reserves and low GI slow ingesting carbs like oats are perfect two hours or so before a workout. For post workout meals choose foods with more of a protein focus to restore glycogen levels and repair muscles. You will still need some carbs and they are still essential after a hard strength session but really try to minimise them in the evenings where possible. Hugh Jackman aka Wolverine follows a diet plan where he doesn't eat any carbs after lunch[13] and so it comes as no surprise to see him looking so ripped in films and on magazine covers if he follows this regime. I tend to take on board energy gels before training sessions if I have not trained after a porridge rich breakfast and I make sure I have thick lentil soup or bean salad or tofu stir fry etc after training as well as protein shakes and bars throughout the day. The overriding thing to remember here is that food is your fuel and you need it to get the most out of your training and your recovery sessions.

6 is the magic number

Food is also linked to your metabolism, the aim is to get the metabolism working fast to keep you lean and the best way to achieve this as any good athlete or sportsperson will tell you is to eat six meals a day. Now before you worry this means six big meals and think "where will I get the time to eat all that?"....it refers to a meal at breakfast, lunch and dinner accompanied with a mid-morning snack, mid-afternoon snack and mid-evening snack. For best effects, Poliquin advocates six to seven meals a day[14]. This type of grazing keeps the metabolism moving. I myself used to be one of those people who only had three meals a day but it played havoc with my digestion. I was leaving it too long between those meals and ignoring hunger pains which caused all sorts of digestive issues. Now by incorporating snacks during the day it curbs hunger. My snacks tend to be protein rich so it feeds the muscle and it reduces the need to eat big meals, all good advantages to be had when trying to get fit fast.

Calorie deficits are your worst enemy

Another really important thing to mention and this tends to be the case for the ladies. Don't skip meals and don't restrict calories to a deficit when you are training. If you take your calorific content down to a level where you are burning off more in the gym, you are not only at a deficit but the body hits that starvation mode where it stores fat to try and protect itself – making it harder for you to lose weight. This makes no sense whatsoever. Stick to regular healthy eating to boost the metabolism.

What about eating out?

Most people tend to worry about following their healthy eating plan when eating out but it doesn't have to be difficult to eat at restaurants. Restaurants are always going to serve steaks, chicken, fish and eggs and for the veggies and vegans you can always get protein from chili dishes and spruce up salads with various beans and vegetables. Most places will accommodate even the fussiest of eaters and this is coming from a Vegan who is also allergic to walnuts and hates mushrooms and onions! If I can do it, so can you. If its lunch time and you are going to train in the afternoon after your meal or at the end of your working day then you can consider pasta or a carb rich meal but in moderation. As mentioned before you need to try and stick away from ingesting carbs of this nature after lunch. I know it's so easy to eat these types of foods in the evening; they are quick and delicious but your body won't thank you for it when the gluten lies in your stomach overnight like glue! Instead try to fill up on juicy vegetables which contain phytochemicals from plants. Phytochemicals present in vegetables contain antioxidants, they reduce inflammation, boost recovery and support your immune system[15] so who wouldn't want some of that?

Beer and Burgers

A quick note on alcohol and fast foods because they do make their way into daily life despite the best laid intentions and plans. Change beer where possible for spirits - your physique will thank you for it and beer bellies are just not a good look! Keep your intake of burgers to a minimum from fast food chains; instead try to cook your own from fresh sources at home. If you have to eat them on the go from fast food chains, drop the buns and just take on the protein from the burger. Remember that things like kebabs may smell nice after a drunken stumble home, but your body will not thank you for putting such rubbish inside it and watch those late night pizzas that are covered in cheese as cheese is high in saturated fats. As mentioned before, if you are going to eat these things, it's better to get it out the way earlier in the day so you can work it off.

If you just can't say no, try to keep it to a sensible minimal treat on a "day off" instead of a daily occurrence!

For those of you interested in what I eat in a normal day here it is :

Breakfast	Bowl of porridge, with blueberries and flaxseed
	Cup of Vanilla Rooibos Tea (decaf)
Mid Morning Snack	Protein shake, banana and a handful of nuts
Lunch	Super Salad - Tofu, lettuce, tomatoes, beetroot, flaxseed, sunflower seed, pumpkin seeds, chai seeds, beans
	Cup of Vanilla Rooibos Tea (decaf)
Mid Afternoon Snack	Protein bar with elderflower still juice
Dinner	Root vegetable roast with edamame beans, pinto beans, aubergine, sugar snap peas, broccoli and cauliflower
	Cup of Vanilla Rooibos Tea (decaf)
Mid Evening Snack	Protein shake or protein bar or Peanut butter on carrots
	Cup of Vanilla Rooibos Tea (decaf)
*During the day I also drink lots of filtered water, especially around training.	

Water, wonderful water

There seems to be no end to the wonders of water. We all know that it's important to drink water during the day and it is mentioned so often in slimming magazines for its wonderful effects on curbing hunger, speeding the metabolism up and keeping skin perfect amongst other things. What if you struggle with water intake as I myself find it the most boring thing ever! My first suggestion is to buy a water filter, it strips out any rubbish in the water (birth control pills, traces of medicines etc), and makes it much cleaner and smoother, delivering a better tasting drink. My second suggestion is to add some cordial (think low/no added sugar versions) but I favour electrolytes - they are like a cheats guide to hydration! They are your essential salts (including sodium, potassium, chloride, bicarbonate, calcium, magnesium, phosphate, sulphate). Just drop one electrolyte tablet in a glass of water and they add flavour as well as boosting hydration levels by replacing essential salts – so a really good one to think about before, during and after any tough workouts where you lose those essential salts.

The wonders of tea

You will have probably worked out now that I like my cups of tea. For as long as I can remember, tea has been in my life in abundance but of latter years I only ever opt for caffeine free so as not to tempt any heart racing moments again. Tea is an absolute gem of a drink, not only does it taste good but researchers at the University College of London found that tea actually lowers cortisol and leads to increased relaxation[16]. During their investigations, the researchers found that cortisol levels had dropped by an average of 47% in a tea drinking group compared with only 27% in a placebo tea group. I have always found it warming and relaxing and with research findings like this, is it any wonder why? Put the kettle on!

Super Foods

There has been a lot said about "Super foods" over the last few years and through trial and error I have come to appreciate which of those foods really are super and now I always aim to have at least two types of those foods from each of the following groups in my cupboards at any one time to make up those super meals that give my body the best chance of looking its best:

Vegetable / Legume	Reasons to love
Broccoli, Cauliflower, Sprouts, Cabbage, Kale (Cruciferous Vegetables)	Rich in Vitamin C to fight against free radicals Contain beta-carotene which helps guard the immune system High in fibre to aid good digestion Rich in Vitamin K to protect bones
Sweet Potatoes	Contain complex carbs that control blood sugar levels Good source of dietary fibre to assist with a healthy digestion system Rich in Vitamins A and C - powerful antioxidants to remove free radicals
Artichokes	Rich in antioxidants that look after the liver A natural diuretic, they aid digestion & improve gallbladder function High in fibre to aid good digestion
Tomatoes	Rich in potassium and Vitamin B they help lower blood pressure and lower cholesterol Rich in Vitamins A and C - powerful antioxidants to remove free radicals The Vitamin A also helps improve vision

Vegetable / Legume	Reasons to love
Beans - Kidney,Pinto, Edamame & Soya	High in protein - essential when trying to build lean muscle mass Rich source of fibre to promote a healthy digestive system High in isoflavones which may promote a healthy heart
Beetroot	Reduces blood pressure to protect the heart Beta cyanin in beetroot can help detox your liver Contains the compound betaine, which enhances the production of the body's natural mood-lifter seratonin
Spinach	Rich in iron to promote strength Vitamin K in Spinach helps keep bones strong Has a high content of Vitamin A which promotes better skin Also has the same benefits as the Cruciferous Vegetables at the top of the table
Watercress	High levels of carotenoids are present in watercress which protects vision Contains potassium to help promote weight loss Has a high calcium content to strengthen the bones and teeth

Fruit	Reasons to love
Avocado	Rich in lutein which helps keep eyes strong
	Good source of potassium, a mineral that helps regulate blood pressure.
	Avocados contain "oleic acid", a monounsaturated fat that may help lower cholesterol
Blueberries, Goji Berries,	Rich in antioxidants to boost the immune system and keep vision healthy
Acai Berries	They help fight abdominal fat
	High fibre content of the berries helps dissolve bad cholesterol to keep the heart healthy
Pomegranate	High in Polyphenols which are very powerful and potent antioxidants that help to protect you from free radicals
	Rich in Vitamin C to help fight off colds
	Contains Vitamin K for healthy bones
Grapefruit	High in enzymes that burn fat and help you lose weight
	Antioxidants present in grapefruit can help reduce cholesterol levels
	Quite high in water content so it assists with hydration
Pineapple	Rich in Bromelain which can assist in improving digestion
	Bromelain has also been found to improve inflammation
Cranberries	Prevents urinary tract infections
	They have anti-inflammatory properties
	Rich in Vitamin C to keep immune system strong

Seed	Reasons to love
Chai Seeds	Balance blood sugar levels and keep you feeling fuller for longer
	Rich in Omega 3 - an essential fatty acid that the body cannot itself produce
	Full of antioxidants to fight against free radicals and keep the immune system strong
Flax Seeds (Linseeds)	Contains lignans and ALA (alpha-linolenic acid) to protect immunity
	Rich in Omega 3 - which can help fight inflammation
	High in soluble and insoluble fibre to keep bowels and digestion healthy
Pumpkin Seeds	High in Zinc which promotes clear skin
	Contain L-tryptophan, a compound naturally effective against depression
	Very good source of magnesium to support muscle and bone health
Sunflower Seeds	Good source of protein and essential amino acids - both essential for muscle growth
	Rich in Vitamin E antioxidants to fight free radicals and protect the immune system
	Contain mono-unsaturated oleic acid which helps lower LDL or "bad cholesterol" and increase HDL or "good cholesterol" in the blood

Nuts	Reasons to love
Macademia	No Cholesterol and high in good fats needed by the body
	High in fibre to keep the digestive system healthy
	Full of phytonutrients to protect our bodies
Almonds	Boost energy due to manganese, copper and riboflavin content
	Rich in nutrients to help the development of the brain
	Vitamin E and monosaturated fats found in almonds are good for the heart
Pistachios	Rich in plant sterols to manage cholesterol effectively
	Contain Carotenoids which are essential for maintaining vision
	One of the highest content of antioxidants
Brazil	Rich in Selenium which helps fight against heart disease and promotes a healthy thyroid
	Contain complete proteins with all the essential amino acids
	Rich in magnesium to keep bones healthy
Walnuts	Contain omega 3 fats which can help protect the arteries
	A good source of melatonin which can helps promote sleep
	Can help fight bad cholesterol

*All nuts are high in protein which is essential for muscle growth.

Peanut butter is also a major part of the famous Abs Diet book which is hailed for its monosaturated heart- healthy fats that also increase testosterone and muscle growth[17]

Meats/Meat Free subs & Poultry	Reasons to love
Soya/Tofu/Quorn	Great meat free alternatives high in protein for muscle growth Good source of isoflavones which can balance hormones Lowers cholesterol
Tuna & Salmon	Rich in essential fatty acids High in protein Rich in Selenium which helps fight against heart disease and promotes a healthy thyroid
Turkey, Chicken & Eggs	Low in fat High in protein Can reduce cholesterol
Beef	Rich in iron to fight off anaemia Contains Zinc which is beneficial for the skin Contains Selenium to keep the heart and thyroid healthy

Herbs, Spices & Oils	Reasons to love
Cinnamon	Vitality booster Controls blood sugar levels Can help boost circulation and ease sickness
Garlic	Can help fight off colds Lowers blood pressure Antiviral content helps fight off allergies
Basil Oil	Rich in antioxidants to fight off free radicals Fights inflammation Contains magnesium to protect bone health
Olive Oil	Contains unsaturated fats that are cholesterol free and can lower cholesterol levels A much healthier alternative to cooking oil Good antioxidant
Cayenne Pepper	One of Beyonce's favourite spices for fat burning Increases the metabolism and promotes digestion Regulates and balances the circulation
Liquorice	Can de-stress and reduce cortisol Can help ease stomach ulcers A natural anti inflammatory

Liquids	Reasons to love
Aloe Vera Juice	Cleanses the colon Eases pains associated with IBS Pain reliever and reduces inflammation
Coconut Milk	Good post workout option rich in medium chain triglycerides – a type of fat that burns readily Rich in phosphorus - an essential nutrient for strong bones High in iron which fights against anaemia
Cranberry Juice	Maintains a healthy urinary tract Natural anti inflammatory Rich in antioxidants to fight against free radicals and keep the immune system strong
Natural Sweeteners (To sweeten porridge)	Made with real fruit to give a natural boost of energy and taste Can be used instead of sugar on pancakes, in porridge and to sweeten curry dishes
Water	The ultimate source of life! Keeps you hydrated and aids in weight loss and can sharpen the metabolism Keeps you feeling fuller for longer

Natural and Organic – it's the only way!

Wherever possible try and buy organic produce – it may be more expensive but it is worth it to avoid the many chemicals now used to treat, develop and grow fruit, vegetables and meats. It goes without saying that fewer chemicals you put into your body, the better because they can turn into toxins that your body then has to deal with – so why put your body through this extra pressure?

Try and extend this philosophy to your toiletries and/or cosmetics regime. We have all too often heard about the potentially damaging effects of parabens and sulphates – so check your product labels and buy wisely. Even the most "natural" looking products can often still contain parabens et al so don't rely on the packaging alone – read the ingredients. The internet is a good place to find the cleaner products as there are quite a few good online "paraben free" stores and now some of the high street retailers are realising they too need to offer these types of products as a matter of choice for men and women. Keep your eyes peeled for "paraben free" statements; products of the like are often grouped together in store.

Some health food stores also offer a good range of more than acceptable shampoos, conditioners, shower gels and cosmetics. There are enough colours, ingredients and flavours in nature to do almost anything with – heading back to older and more traditional pre-war methods are often the cleanest and safest ways to live! Go paraben free – your body will thank you for it.

Have a day off!

It is important not to totally deny the body what it craves, as we all know it just makes us want it even more! So make sure you build in a day each week where you can reward yourself with that pizza or cookie or bag of crisps if you need to. Some athletes believe in a carb re-feed one day a week as it boosts energy. Again see how your body reacts but don't go overboard on that day otherwise all your hard work will start to slide! Timothy Ferris, author of the 4 Hour Body, advocates carb re-feeding and believed it helped him achieve and develop his muscular physique[18].

Summary

- There are an astounding number of successful vegan athletes – it's time to join them!
- Understand the many benefits of plant based proteins, they are full of goodness and healthy nutrition - perfect for your body development plan.
- High protein diets are very important to build and also repair muscle in the body.
- Cut down on simple carbs and try not to eat any after lunch unless you are training in the afternoon, where carbs are needed prior to your workout for energy and endurance.
- There are good carbs out there – sweet potato, brown rice and porridge being good examples.
- Think 6-7 meals a day to keep your metabolism revving.
- Don't be tempted to skip meals or have a calorie deficit both are counterproductive and a total waste of time.
- Remain on track when eating out, just remember what you are trying to achieve.
- Water is essential in the world of fitness; it will keep you hydrated, curb hunger and assist in weight loss.
- Drink tea to de-stress; its research proven to reduce cortisol levels.
- Stock up on Super Foods – use as many items as possible throughout the week.
- Buy organic foods were possible and extend this to buying clean, chemical free toiletries. Buy clean....feel clean!
- Give yourself a day off every now and again and consider carb re-feeds– don't go all Sergeant Strict 100% of the time, it will drive you mad!
- Don't forget about your good fats – found in avocados, seeds & nuts.

CHAPTER 3 - SUPPLEMENTS

Get acquainted with Vitamins

It is amazing how many people I have met who complain they are not achieving what they want in the gym despite putting the time in or if they are working out quite well, they complain of other problems like aches, pains, tiredness, slow recovery or many other weird and wonderful complaints. It comes as no surprise when doing a little bit of digging with these people to find out they have never taken a vitamin tablet in their life and they seem put off by supplements as they are convinced they get everything they need from their diet. There within lies one of the biggest problems and I always give the advice to bring supplements into your life, even if it is just one multi vitamin per day to keep the immune system strong and help you get through the day.

Vitamins are your body's best friend

There are a whole raft of reasons as to why I recommend you take supplements, but the main pivot around the fact that today's food does not contain all the necessary nutrients for you to be in tip top form, as they are heavily polluted with all sorts of chemicals unless you buy 100% organic and the foods that do contain vitamins are digested by your body and then depart from your body at a fairly quick rate, so it is essential to top up and consume the vitamins and minerals that you may be low or deficient in. If you want to get a little more scientific about this, you can go and have a vitamin/mineral deficiency test at your nearest natural health practice. I make a few visits here during the year to test three things – firstly the food sensitivity test to make sure my food choices align with what my digestive system needs. Secondly to test my levels of vitamins and minerals and thirdly to test hormone levels, as they need to be balanced for both males and females if you want to get the most from your training.

Where to start

So where do you start in order to know what you are looking for? It all starts with thinking about what you want to achieve – now we all want to protect our bones, preserve our muscular skeleton system, improve our recovery and keep our joints supple. These are all really big factors in making sure we get the most from our workouts so they need to be covered off with the right supplements. On the same front we don't want coughs and colds to interrupt our training regimes and we also want to feel strong and have enough energy to get ourselves to the gym, so these too are important areas to look at. Natural vitamins can be sourced from your local health store which may help with all of the above, it's as easy as that and it's not going to make you look like a body builder and it won't make you grow a "bruisers beard" – result!!

Coming up next is a list of what I take in a normal day – it looks a lot but I feel great, I have no side effects and I sleep like a baby so here is what I take and a brief look at why I take it:

Supplement	Rationale for taking	Daily Dosage	Time of the day taken
Vegan multivitmin & mineral	Selection of vitamins and minerals to keep my RDA at its max	1	Breakfast
Kelp 300g	Contains iodine which my diet is low in Regulates the metabolism Maintains healthy skin	1	Breakfast

Supplement	Rationale for taking	Daily Dosage	Time of the day taken
Bio Carnitine 250mg	Helps in the body's production of energy Helps maintain a healthy heart and skeletal muscle	1	Breakfast
Vegetarian Glucosomine Hydrochloride 1500mg	Helps maintain healthy joints and cartilage	1	Breakfast
Vitamin C 1000mg	Keeps the immune system strong High in antioxidants to fight against free radicals	1	Breakfast
Magnesium 250mg	Supports bone and muscle health Assists in restful sleep	1	Breakfast
Calcium with Vit D 600mg	Supports the maintenance of healthy bone density Vitamin D helps calcium intake	2	Breakfast
Zinc 25mg	Protects immune system Keeps spots at bay!	1	Evening
Compose Rehamania & Schisandra	Keeps stress away Contains Chinese herbs that lower cortisol	4	2 with Lunch 2 with Dinner
USN Power Punch BCAA drink	Muscle recovery, repair and lean muscle growth	2 scoops in 500ml water	Before, during & after workouts

A good starting point would be to have a look at the supplements mentioned on the previous page as these are very comprehensive and general for what you will be trying to achieve fitness wise. Give some of them a go – do this for a month and I am sure you will see big differences in strength, energy, a reduction in colds and an all-round better immune system. Experiment and see what works for you – your body will thank you for it.

It's all about routine

Now on first glance, you may think that I take a lot of supplements, but the majority of them are taken before breakfast in the morning so I do not have to carry around that many pills during the day. Think "routine and repetition" and you will soon get into the swing of things. I now just class them as part of meal times so I don't forget.

Branched Chain Amino Acids

One particular supplement I want to talk about in isolation is that of *Branched Chain Amino Acids*. BCAA are a group of 3 amino acids; Leucine, Isoleucine and Valine and in tablet form they are the perfect gym buddies for anyone who is lifting weights, as they protect muscle mass and improve recovery time immeasurably whilst offering support for the immune defence system. Charles Poliquin is a big crusader of BCAAs and has written numerous articles on their benefits[19]. Our bodies will confiscate our amino acids and use them when needed for energy instead of muscle building and this sometimes explains why you may not see spectacular changes in your muscle growth when training hard with weights. Branched chain amino acids are very important in the muscle building process and if you supplement during your workout there will not be a need for your body to scavenge them from your muscle tissue and you will have provided an optimum state for regrowth of muscle tissue[20]. You will essentially be stopping the needless breakdown of precious muscle tissue for energy purposes which is a great help when trying to achieve that athletic look. Taking BCAA increases the release of anabolic (regenerative) hormones and decreases the amount of catabolic (degenerative) hormones. In a more anabolic environment our bodies will release insulin and cut back on producing cortisol – which is another reason to take it, as anything that reduces cortisol helps to eliminate stresses that can cause fat.

Charles Poliquin Protocols

In addition to the "staple diet" of vitamins and minerals mentioned above I also try various protocols during the year, most of which operate on the basis of Charles Poliquin's teachings and again can be seen in the table below:

PROTOCOL 1			
Product	Rationale	Daily dosage	Time of the day taken
Poliquin Fenuplex	Supports healthy glucose metabolism	3-6	Before Breakfast, Lunch & Dinner
Poliquin Insulinomics	Supports healthy insulin function (good if you consume high carbs)	3-6	Before Breakfast, Lunch & Dinner

PROTOCOL 2			
Product	Rationale	Daily dosage	Time of the day taken
Poliquin Insulinomics	Supports healthy insulin function (good if you consume high carbs)	3-6	Before Breakfast, Lunch & Dinner
Poliquin Glucose Disposal PX	Botanic herbs optimise blood sugar control	3-6	Before Breakfast, Lunch & Dinner
PROTOCOL 3			
Product	Rationale	Daily dosage	Time of the day taken
Nutri DIM	Oestrogen balance and metabolic clearing	6	2 at Breakfast, Lunch & Dinner
Poliquin Primal Fibre	Promotes a healthy intestinal function	2 tablespoons	3 at Breakfast & Dinner
Poliquin Calcium D Glucarate	Detoxifies oestrogens	3-6	1 glass before Breakfast & Dinner

*Vegans/Vegetarians please note, any Poliquin supplements that are packed in a gelatine shell, I buy a supply of gelatine free capsules that I repack them in – you can get them from your local health food store or online.

The protocols were employed particularly for me to deal with two areas:

1. Original overindulgence of carbohydrates – Being a vegan makes it hard to avoid carbs as they are high in pasta, rice, potatoes, cereals and bread. I stripped those out of my diet other than before a training session, but in the phase of carb reduction I found that taking Protocol 1 and switching it with Protocol 2 was excellent. It also assisted in a lowering of body fat and in particular stripping down the supra-iliac (oblique) site to its lowest point with a 35% reduction in this site (Poliquin™ BioSignature modulation result). I now dip in and out of the protocols whenever I feel I need them most during the year.

2. Balancing oestrogens – Soya is a part of my diet but it can sometimes promote bad oestrogens and I also had a hormone level test carried out at Wilmslow Health Practice that also showed the same thing so Protocol 3 was perfect for eradicating this. I do this for one or two months a year max for best results.

Creatine – To take or not to take?

Found in fish and meats but also in our muscle cells, Creatine is used to fuel movement in the muscles. Creatine monohydrate (a synthetic form of Creatine) is one of the most researched and purchased sports nutrition products in the world and its worth mentioning in brief so that you understand what it is and whether you will benefit from it. In a study undertaken on fifteen female university crew team members, Stout et al (1999) found that Creatine delayed the onset of neuromuscular fatigue[21]. This remains one of the main reasons people take Creatine – basically in order to workout longer and this relates to lifting weights for longer or running for longer. I take Creatine during the winter; it has definitely helped me on the longer cross country running as I don't feel as tired when taking it. I also find if I have hit a plateau in the weights game and just need a little extra oomph it helps me through that. I don't do anything as scientific as loading on and off Creatine, but many gym-goers tend to operate that way for maximum effect. Have a think if there could be a use for this supplement in your fitness regime and try it out whilst measuring your progress; you will soon know if it works for you but it definitely does work for me.

Friendly fats

Fats get a lot of bad press and whenever you see the word "fat", you tend to have a negative connotation with it, but there are some fats in foods and supplements that are healthy, friendly fats that will help you with your fitness goals. These are referred to as the Essential Fats or Essential Fatty Acids (EFA's) - commonly known as Omega 3 and Omega 6. These fats cannot be manufactured in the body, they have to be taken either via diet or supplementation. In terms of diet, the kind of botanical foods that you need to be eating to increase your EFA's are soy, flaxseed, avocados, chai, sunflower and sesame seeds. Animal sources include fish, beef and eggs. Research has shown that EFAs increase bone mineral density[22], reduce inflammation[23], and can also help with signs of depression[24]. If you struggle to get these food groups into your diet, or if you are keen like me to up your dosage of EFA's, the best option is to select a supplement that delivers it for you – Flaxseed Oil in capsules is a good choice and they are widely available from all good health food stores. I also make sure I sprinkle those super seeds in salads, soups and porridge too.

L Carnitine

There are quite a lot of supplements on the market that claim to burn fat away. Some take the route of being made with ingredients that curb the appetite whilst others contain ingredients that have been found to metabolise fat in the body. After trying quite a lot over the years I have found that disappointingly the majority contain caffeine – normally from green tea extract which again is a favourite in the slimming world. Being too caffeine sensitive, and not wanting to get the heart racing, shaky feelings, I looked and tested multiple alternatives and L Carnitine and Chromium have been the best for me in terms of overall effectiveness. In 1992, Kaats found that these two ingredients can reduce body weight, reduce body fat but protect body mass whilst also increasing the metabolic rate and decreasing cholesterol[25]. L Carnitine has not only been linked to weight loss but also to increased fitness performance with particular reference to better power output and less lactic acid build ups[26]. If you are struggling to shift those final few pounds give a fat burner like L Carnitine a go – it could just be the final piece of puzzle that pushes you further to your dream physique.

> Grapefruit is a natural fat burner you can incorporate into your diet. Take half with lunch and the other half with dinner. Avoid taking at breakfast as it can interfere with supplements and/or medication.

Gathering the knowledge made easy

The great thing about the world of supplements is that no matter how confusing you may think it is – it does happen to be a constant talking point in magazines that cover health and fitness, so you can start by reading a few of those magazines that you may already buy and make some notes on supplements that seem to be rich in elements that you want to increase. The other nice thing about this industry is that it is absolutely packed with specialists - the shop owners and workers both in the independent and multiple health food chains. If you walk into your nearest health food store and explain to the staff what you are looking for, you will be faced with the most helpful of characters who can tell you about every healing herb and every benefit of any vitamins and minerals.

Give others the good news

Before you know it, you will be totally empowered with this information and you'll smile and remember this when you are taking your tablets and a friend or family member asks you what you are taking and why! I am sure you will enjoy passing on your knowledge with them and many others will naturally follow your lead as you will be looking fabulous after being on those essential supplements!

Alternative therapies

Inside the health food stores are also a range of other interesting products that you will no doubt be attracted to – some of my favourites both in terms of past times and also effective results include: Aromatherapy, Crystal Healing, the power of Flower Oils (Bach's Flower Remedy in particular) and Homeopathy. Have a read around these subjects, most of which can help relax and reduce stress as well as treating some minor medical conditions. It's a whole new world and I challenge you not to fall in love with it!

Summary

- It's time to know your supplements!
- Take BCAAs before, during and after exercise
- Consider getting a vitamin/mineral deficiency test.
- Creatine can make you stronger for longer!
- Keep your EFA's up for optimum performance.
- Burn that fat away with L Carnitine – get shredded!
- Understand your ailments and don't be afraid to self-treat with the wonderful herbs and vitamins out there.
- Take advantage of the knowledge that the health food shops have – ask for help.
- Immerse yourself with the information on vitamins/minerals/supplements and empower others.
- Think about other alternative treatments to further reduce any stress levels.

CHAPTER 4 – STATE OF MIND

Laugh and the world laughs with you

"Laughing policeman", "Foghorn Gawthorne", "Gigglebot" –
I could go on and mention some more of the colourful names
I have collected from family and friends over the years, of which
there are many but these are just a few that home in on my
constant ability to guffaw or "laugh like a sea lion" as one of my
friends describes it. The reason I mention this is because
laughing is of course important - it is the backbone of positivity.
It is no coincidence that the Japanese proverb "Time spent
laughing is time spent with the gods" is one of my favourite
sayings. I have never met anyone who seems to laugh as much as
I do and even that I find quite amusing, but the one thing I do
know is that it has helped me so much in life to be this way and
it's always been natural. It comes as a bonus for me to learn that
laughter reduces stress hormones epinephrine and cortisol[27].
Everything seems quite funny in my world but this also has a
real good advantage as it keeps stress at bay so it is another
important part of the puzzle to stay happy and be positive.
I am constantly reading about laughter and its effects, recently
I have seen laughter yoga classes taking place in China on TV
where people meet in a park and practise the art of laughing with
yoga - what a perfect combination for happiness and relaxation!
I have also learned that laughter reduces the firmness of arteries,
lessening the risk of heart problems[28]. It's all good stuff so laugh
for happiness and healthiness! Watch your favourite comedian,
surround yourself with people who make you laugh; the lighter
your mood, the lighter your weight is likely to be!

Positivity & Motivation

Achieving your ideal body starts with the obvious in the gym and continues on the tangible trail with changes to diet and supplementation but perhaps one of the most overlooked and difficult to manage quadrants is that of the intangible - the mind. It is essential that your mind is in a receptive state to training and that it understands what you need to do, when you need to do it, how you should do it and most importantly how you can do it if you are not feeling very motivated.

Motivation starts with positivity – you have to see the goal, you have to be aware of what it is you want to achieve and then you have to remain in that mind-set, locking on to that target if you are serious about improving your body, your diet, your fitness levels and your overall health.

Ok so let's start with a major positive – you have purchased or acquired this book – by the very nature of the topic it has been bought or borrowed with intention and that intention is to make a positive change, to make you feel better about yourself, to enable you to live a "guilt free" life – the latter in regards to food consumption and time spent in the gym. A positive root of this nature is only ever going to be destined to grow and soon enough you will start to feel proud as you grow with it.

There is just no time!

Working out, eating healthy and taking supplements all require management – they require management in terms of time, they also need to be planned in terms of quantity practised/consumed and of course budget management. For the purpose of getting the best of this chapter, I will assume that you have a gym membership or access to fitness equipment and it will also be assumed that vitamin/mineral protocols are all affordable and managed. This leaves the way we work out and the food we eat – these two important aspects are both seriously compromised by one thing – Time.

Busy working schedules, manic social plans, childcare quandaries and other family commitments are unfortunately the norm for most people. The first trick here is to just purely acknowledge them. I find it quite beneficial to work from a Time/System which is similar to a Filofax but offers more planning dimensions. Each week I list the appointments and business meetings and anything that requires me to be in a different place or anything that upsets my normal routine gets listed. Then this leaves potential gaps – gaps in which you can plan your training sessions effectively and even if you have minimal time you can always slot in a fat torching high interval session – it may only be 20 minutes but boy you will feel like you have worked out for days after it and it's a great conditioning technique. So what I am alluding to say is that *there is no excuse!* Those four words are said time and time again by personal trainers all over the world, they are basic but they are true. It makes your life so much easier if on a Sunday evening you put aside five minutes of your time to plan out how your forthcoming week will look. Where and when you will work out will soon become second nature once you do this a few times. It will also help to reduce those all-important cortisol levels as you will be less stressed throughout the week trying to guess when you are going to work out and exactly what it is you are doing each session.

Finding the positives from the unexpected

For the majority of time, your plan will work out well, but on the odd occasion that something unexpected happens and interrupts your training schedule try to find the positive in it – could you for example benefit from an extra days rest if you can't get away to train or if you don't have as much time as originally planned to train could you cut down your training time and do a fast and furious workout that would condition your overall body in a much more beneficial way than that long hard slog on a cardio machine? Whichever way you look at it start to find those positives because they are there and this is something that as a self-confessed multiple year fitness fanatic, I found to be one of the most important, effective and advantageous things to practise. It is the hardest pill to swallow when you are training for a third of the time you used to with your cardio and this is where training your mind to accept the situation is key.

Mind Mapping for mind clarity

Another good way to plan out your weeks or indeed anything you are working on is the use of Mind Mapping created by Tony Buzan[29]. Mind Mapping is a very easy way of getting everything down on a diagram so you can understand all the effects and the influences. This is a very good way to clear out the mind too! See the next page for a mind map on achieving dream body status.

Plan the food shopping

Once you have planned your week out, you can then move on to think about what types of food you will need in the house or with you at work to power your workouts and fuel those all-important recovery periods to keep you in tip-top shape. You can plan out your shopping in the areas of carbs and proteins to complement your training schedule. Again this will make life a lot easier for you as you can plan the shopping around it and not have the excuse of being without the right ingredients or the right foods.

It will also be the basis for you to understand which foods work well with your training and when to consume them – essential and again after a little investigation it will become natural to

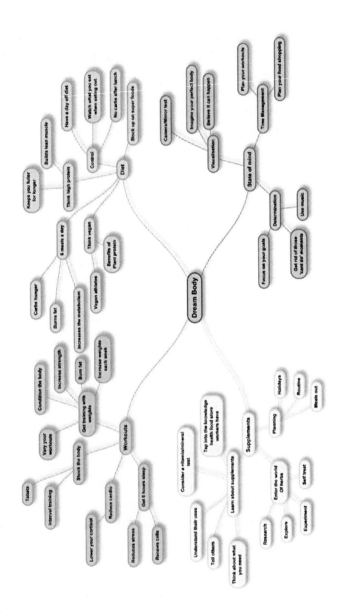

Mind Map – How to achieve the dream body

shop this way! It also makes for interesting times as your shopping becomes a workout as you dart round filling up on proteins then carbs etc., choosing not to follow the normal trail in the supermarket and instead moving freely wherever your fitness goals lead you. Whilst you shimmy across the supermarket aisles why not tense your abs for ten seconds then release, then do the same with your butt – repeat this ten times over and you have just done a mini fat shredding workout whilst on the move and to nobody's knowledge!

Keeping the focus at the gym

So you are now equipped at managing your time and diet, what's next? It's on to the actual workouts themselves and how you think and feel about them. When you are in the gym the aim is to keep focused and driven no matter whether you are there for stretching, remedial work, concentrated body weights or cardio. You need to know what it is you are hoping to achieve from your time (which is precious) in the gym, you need to record the feeling you have when you have worked out hard – record what it feels like at that point in time when you deserve to have a big smile painted on your face. Capturing that feeling and using it as the end point will drive you nicely through the toughest of workouts.

Can't do moments

Whilst you are actually at the gym or about to workout at home or maybe go for a run, you will encounter some famous and well known "can't do" moments, here are just a few of them:

- *I can't lift this weight, it is too heavy for me*
- *I can't run any further, I am totally depleted of all drive*
- *I can't do this many reps or circuits, I just run out of energy*

- *I can't go any faster or add any more resistance to this bike*
- *I can't do any more intervals without longer recovery periods*

Write down your most used "can't do" moments and then take them one by one and try and attack them as if you were your own personal trainer – what would your trainer say, would he say something like "come on you only have to give it your all for few more seconds", or perhaps she would say "two more reps then a lovely long rest" – what I am trying to highlight here is that you yourself are a powerful tool and when you don't have access to a trainer, you can use your own methods of encouragement – you can motivate yourself just as much as any trainer but you have to be driven by your overall goal and once that is clear in your head this all becomes so much easier.

Be your own motivator

Mental preparation will make your workouts seem more intense but oh so worthwhile. One of the best and easiest methods of utilising this psyche is to have "secret" motivational conversations with yourself although sometimes you do see the odd word coming out of my mouth if I am really using everything I have on my last rep of an exercise, so don't beat yourself up if that happens just keep it clean if others are about!

The magic of music

Another great tool thanks to the legendary Steve Jobs is the I Pod – get your most motivational playlists banging out, feel the beat, use the energy and lose yourself in this zone and you will be surprised how far you can run, or how much you can lift when listing to the Rocky Soundtrack which is a prerequisite for all fitness followers! Use whatever music works for you – my PT James uses Heavy Rock which I could not listen to for one second, but it works well for him! I favour high energy dance tracks but occasionally some slow vocals when the mood suits. The key is to home in on the genres that work for you and like your workouts you need to keep refreshing your playlists because they will soon become boring and it can reach a level where it demotivates you as you seek a tune you have not heard for a while only to realise that you have listened to your I pod that much you have worked your way through it and back in the last 5 days! Keep it fresh – it will keep you on track with your fitness sessions and it will keep your mind-set at the gym nice and fresh and positive too.

Visualisation

Now on to those days where you just don't feel like dragging your butt off the sofa or out of bed to get to the gym or do a training session - this will all become a thing of the past once you walk yourself through the trees of visualisation. If you want to immerse yourself in this method, one of the best books to read on it is the best-selling book "The Secret" by Rhonda Byrne[30]. The Secret is a fabulous book that looks at how you can achieve overall happiness, if you believe it and you actually see it before it happens. You need to have a think about what your ideal body would look like, where would the curves be? Where would you look ripped? How much weight will you have lost from your stomach? How toned would your arms look?

Once you have that overall body image in your mind now give thought to how you would dress it, would you get into that suit now the beer belly has gone?, Would you wear figure hugging jogging pants to show off your toned butt?, Would you don the latest designer vest to show how ripped your biceps look?

Would you finally be able to fit into those dream jeans, that dream dress?....are you are getting the picture? Keep this image at the forefront of your mind and whenever your falter or start to struggle for motivation, bring it to life and remember that your workouts are scheduled to get you there or for those who are already there, to keep you there!

Here's the weird bit, you won't need this once you achieve your ideal body as you will be aware of all this and all you have to do is look in the mirror and think about the fact that you have worked hard to get where you are and it's up to you to keep working hard (in moderation) to keep it.

Monitor your hard work and progress

Take pictures of yourself along your journey and look back over them to notice the differences – this is a really good way to work out what works for you and what makes you look your best. All you have to do for this is take a few pictures with your mobile phone in front of the mirror and try and repeat the pose each month to allow you to identify the differences. This way you can recall what you were eating at the time and how you were working out if you have kept a rough diary of exercise sessions and meals (not many people have time to do this but it will help you identify the most effective training methods). Then you will have a small collection of pictures that correspond with any changes. If you want to take this one step further, get your body fat measured every month or so with callipers (digital machines are not accurate) and then you will begin to understand what 20% body fat actually looks like. Search for your nearest Poliquin certified Biosignature instructor for accurate readings. Alternatively if you have a personal trainer you can ask if they can do this and if they can't, you will easily find some local sports colleges with the facilities.

Summary

- Positivity – harness the power of smiles, laughter and happiness – it reduces the stress hormones.
- Determination – stay focused, be aware of your goals at all times.
- Time Management – plan your workouts, your food requirements, make your diary work for you.
- Embrace the unexpected –consider having a day of extra rest if you have to work late or minimise your time in the gym with a 20 minute fat torching circuit.
- Mind Map – it will clear the clutter from your mind.
- Get over your "can't do's" – use motivation tricks – use self-talking and music that makes you tap your feet.
- Be your own personal trainer –push yourself past the comfortable zone.
- Visualisation – think of that perfect body – imagine how good it looks or look at yourself in the mirror if you are already there and think about what you need to do to maintain it.
- Monitor your hard work - practise the camera-mirror test so you have results to monitor.

Final Thoughts

Now before you put the book down I want you to remember that your dream physique is going to be a really interesting and enjoyable journey and I am sure you will find different ways and methods that work for you as you move along the journey.

I urge and encourage you to incorporate any new routines that work well into your program, as a varied workout is always best. I still buy the odd book and the odd magazine to see if there are any new or different exercises I can put into my routines – as it's all about change and keeping it fresh. The internet is a hive of information in the world of fitness. I often print off new training sessions to try them out and this keeps my training in a constant moving platform for better effects. You can do this in between your 12 or 16 week cycles, you may choose to add in some strength training or volume training or a workout from your favourite fitness magazine. You won't go wrong by following it for no more than 4 weeks then changing on to a different workout and remember when you finally do go back to the start, you will be stronger and so you will be working harder all the time, pushing yourself to new limits so you continue to get the results you really want to see.

The book is as near as you are going to get to a prescription that delivers what you want, so enjoy yourself as you start the journey. You will feel in control once you get your head around the four quadrants of working out, diet, supplements and your state of mind - it will all slot into place.

It will take a little time for you to get used to your new regime but you will get there and even if at the very least this book has inspired you to just merely put more weights sessions into your week, then that is a major win as I am sure you will see visible results and I guarantee you will want to build on that in the other quadrants to see even better results moving forward.

Happy training, happy eating, happy supplementing, happy thoughts!

Lisa

References

1. Alpert, K. (2009), Getting maximum Results Part I: Alternatives to Aerobics. Six Reasons why Aerobic work is counterproductive. http://www.charlespoliquin.com/ArticlesMultimedia/Articles/Article/25/Getting_Maximum_Results_Part_I_-_Alternatives_to_A.aspx

2. Polilquin, C. (2011), How to counter the many negative effects of aerobic training. http://www.charlespoliquin.com/ArticlesMultimedia/Articles/Article/734/How_to_Counter_The_Many_Negatives_of_Aerobic_Train.aspx

3. Talbott, S.M. (2002), The Cortisol Connection – Why stress makes you fat and ruins your health and what you can do about it, 1st edition, Hunter House Inc Publishers.

4. Nybo, L et al. (2010), High-intensity training versus traditional exercise interventions for promoting health. Medicine and science in sports and exercise, 2010 Oct; 42(10):1951-8. Department of Exercise and Sport Sciences, University of Copenhagen, Copenhagen, Denmark.

5. Price, D. (2011), Tabata Training. http://articles.muscletalk.co.uk/article-tabata-training.aspx

6. Sundell, J. (2011), Resistance Training Is an Effective Tool against Metabolic and Frailty Syndromes. Advances in Preventative Medicine, 2011; 2011:984683. Epub 2010 Dec 13. Department of Medicine, University of Turku, Finland.

7. George, J.W. et al (2006) The effects of active release technique on hamstring flexibility: a pilot study, Journal of

Manipulative and Physiological Therapeutics, Volume: 29, Issue: 3, Pages: 224-227.

8. Taheri, Dr. S (2010), Sleep yourself skinny: It's not only leaving us shattered and ill. Experts say too little shut-eye is making us fat. Daily Mail, 15th Feb 2010. Flic Everett. http://www.dailymail.co.uk/femail/article-1250992/Sleep-skinny-Its-leaving-shattered-ill-Experts-say-little-shut-eye-making-fat.html

9. Van Cauter, E. (2010), Sleep yourself skinny: It's not only leaving us shattered and ill. Experts say too little shut-eye is making us fat. Daily Mail, 15th Feb 2010. Flic Everett. http://www.dailymail.co.uk/femail/article-1250992/Sleep-skinny-Its-leaving-shattered-ill-Experts-say-little-shut-eye-making-fat.html

10. Hamilton, S.F & Antonio, J. (2004), Fast Track: Training and Nutrition Secrets from Americas top Female Runner, Rodale Inc Publishing.

11. Layman, D.K. (2004), Protein quantity and quality at levels above the RDA improves adult weight loss. Journal of the American College of Nutrition, 2004 Dec; 23(6 Suppl):631S-636S.

12. Antonio J, at al. (2008), Essentials of Sports Nutrition and Supplements. *International Society of Sports Nutrition.* Humana Press 2008.

13. Beard, J. (2009), The Mirror. http://www.mirror.co.uk/celebs/celebs-on-sunday/2009/05/10/hugh-jackman-i-want-people-to-think-i-could-rip-their-head-off-115875-21334554/

14. Poliquin, C. (2009), The Protein Goal Diet. A brief description of Charles protein goal system for fat loss. http://www.charlespoliquin.com/ArticlesMultimedia/Articles/Article/113/The_Protein_Goal_Diet.aspx

15. De La Rosa, L.A. (2009), Fruit and Vegetable Phytochemicals: Chemistry, Nutritional Value and Stability, 1st edition, Wiley-Blackwell Publishing.

16. Steptoe, A et al. (2006), The effects of tea on psychophysiological stress responsivity and post stress recovery: a randomised double-blind trial. Phychopharmacology 190: 81-89, University of College London

17. Zinczenko, D. (2004), The Abs Diet, Rodale Inc Publishing.

18. Ferris, T. (2010), The 4-Hour Body, An uncommon guide to rapid fat loss, incredible sex and becoming superhuman. Random House Group Publishing.

19. Poliquin, C. (2011), The Benefits of BCAA's: 10 Quick Tips and Detailed Research. http://www.charlespoliquin. com/ArticlesMultimedia/Articles/Article/654/The_Benefit s_of_BCAAs_10_Quick_Tips_and_Detailed_R.aspx

20. Muscle Marketing USA World Product Booklet: Amino Acids. The Building Blocks of Protein, P18.

21. Stout et al. (1999)"Effect of creatine loading on neuromuscular fatigue threshold." Journal of American Physiology 88: 109-112. http://jap.physiology.org/content/88/1/109.full

22. Hogstrom M at al. (2007), n-3 Fatty acids are positively associated with peak bone mineral density and bone accrual in healthy men: the NO2 Study. Am J Clin Nutr. 2007; 85(3):803-7.

23. Mori TA & Beilin LJ. (2004), Omega-3 fatty acids and inflammation. Curr Atheroscler Rep. 2004;6(6):461-7. School of Medicine and Pharmacology—Royal Perth Hospital Unit, The University of Western Australia, Medical Research Foundation Building, Perth, Western Australia 6847, Australia.

24. Bourre JM. (2005), Dietary Omega-3 Fatty Acids and Psychiatry: Mood, Behaviour, Stress, Depression, Dementia and Ageing. J Nutr Health Ageing. 2005; 9 (1):31-38.

25. Kaats, Gilbert R, et al. (1992), "The short-term therapeutic efficacy of treating obesity with a plan of improved nutrition and moderate caloric restriction," Current Therapeutic Research Vol. 51, No. 2 (Feb 1992): 261-274.

26. Vecchiet, L, et al. (1990), "Influence of L-carnitine administration on maximal physical exercise," European Journal of Applied Physiology 61 (1990): 486-490.

27. Scott, E. (2011), The stress management and health benefits of laughter. http://stress.about.com/od/stresshealth/a/laughter.htm

28. Vlachopoulos, C et al. (2009), The Official Journal of the American Psychosomatic Society Volume 71 Number 4, Psychosomatic Medicine Journal of Biobehavioral Medicine. Divergent Effects of Laughter and Mental Stress on Arterial Stiffness and Central Hemodynamics, p446.

29. Buzan, T. (2010), The Mind Map Book: Unlock your creativity, boost your memory, change your life, BBC Active.

30. Byrne, R. (2006), The Secret, Simon & Schuster UK Ltd Publishing.

Bibliography &
Further Reading Resources

1body4life (Active Release Techniques) http://www.1body4life.
co.uk/

Active Release Technique http://www.activerelease.com/

Bach's Flower Information http://www.bachcentre.com/centre/
remedies.htm

Buav http://www.buav.org/

Freedman, R & Barnouin, K. (2005), Skinny Bitch, Running
Press Book Publishers.

Laughter Yoga Information http://www.laughteryoga.org/

Meat Free Mondays www.meatfreemondays.com

Morton, D. (2011), Mens Health Muscle Manual, Summer
2011, Part 1, Rodale Publishing.

My Pure (Paraben Free products) www.mypure.co.uk

Phytochemicals Information http://www.phytochemicals.info/

Price, R.C. (2005), The Ultimate Guide to Weight Training for
Running, Second Edition.

Primal Health Personal Trainers http://www.primalhealthfitness.
co.uk/